Keto Living For The Super Busy
Eat to Lose Weight

Rick Elliott

Legal & Disclaimer

The information contained in this book and its contents is not designed to replace or take the place of any form of medical or professional advice; and is not meant to replace the need for independent medical, financial, legal or other professional advice or services, as may be required. The content and information in this book has been provided for educational and entertainment purposes only.

The content and information contained in this book has been compiled from sources deemed reliable, and it is accurate to the best of the Author's knowledge, information and belief. However, the Author cannot guarantee its accuracy and validity and cannot be held liable for any errors and/or omissions. Further, changes are periodically made to this book as and when needed. Where appropriate and/or necessary, you must consult a professional (including but not limited to your doctor, attorney, financial advisor or such other professional advisor) before using any of the suggested remedies, techniques, or information in this book.

Upon using the contents and information contained in this book, you agree to hold harmless the Author from and against any damages, costs, and expenses, including any legal fees potentially resulting from the application of any of the information provided by this book. This disclaimer applies to any loss, damages or injury caused by the use and application, whether directly or indirectly, of any advice or information presented, whether for breach of contract, tort, negligence, personal injury, criminal intent, or under any other cause of action.

You agree to accept all risks of using the information presented inside this book.

You agree that by continuing to read this book, where appropriate and/or necessary, you shall consult a professional (including but not limited to your doctor, attorney, or financial advisor or such other advisor as needed) before using any of the suggested remedies, techniques, or information in this book.

Legal & Disclaimer

The information contained in this book and its contents is not designed to replace or take the place of any form of medical or professional advice; and is not meant to replace the need for independent medical, financial, legal or other professional advice or services, as may be required. The content and information in this book has been provided for educational and entertainment purposes only.

Contents

Introduction

Health problems around the world have been largely caused by unhealthy lifestyles. There are so many different weight loss programs and diets out there, all touting to make you slimmer, healthier, if you choose to adopt their methods.

The ketogenic diet must not be totally alien to you. It's the latest 'revolutionary' diet craze to hit us in recent memory. In case you aren't familiar with the keto diet, here's a rundown. In most diets, the focus is primarily on lowering fat consumption. "Don't eat fatty food! It'll make you fat!" This sounds so obvious, but recent studies have shown that if you want to shed fat fast, you must instead increase your fat intake and instead, limit your cabs intake. This is essentially what the ketogenic diet is all about.

In a Ketogenic diet, the focus is on reducing carbs since carbs are considered the main source of fuel for the human body. You might wonder if you can even exercise while on a restricted carb diet. You need to keep in mind that exercise is still possible and can bring you closer to the fulfillment of your weight loss goals.

When it comes to weight loss, it's a common notion that you need to eat less and exercise more. However, this traditional viewpoint has grown obsolete. If you really want to see a leaner body while losing weight, you need to consider what you eat. One should pay more attention to a quality diet rather than only considering the quantity of consumption

In this book , you will be introduced and guided to experience the myriads of health benefits you can get while on a Ketogenic Diet. It is a motivational process to encourage you towards a shift in your present dietary lifestyle.

Healthy ways must be incorporated into your daily lifestyle to become a habit, we do not advocate yo-yo fad diets that will disappear in a short period of time, in favor of yet another fangled new diet.

Also, this book includes several sample Diet meal plans with mouth-watering dishes which will not only taste good but gives your body a well-balanced ketogenic diet.

Chapter 1: The Science of Ketosis

The ketogenic diet cannot be labeled as a new discovery. In fact, it has existed in various forms and similarities from other diet plans such as the Atkin's, Paleo and South Beach diets.

To begin with, understand that ketogenic diet has three types: 1) The Standard Ketogenic Diet; 2) the Cyclical Ketogenic Diet; and 3) the Targeted Ketogenic Diet. All three are co-related but differ only in terms of control and timing of the carbohydrate consumption.

As defined, the ketogenic diet is a diet that makes one's body undergo the process called "ketosis." During this process, the body draws energy from burned fats instead of carbohydrates. Therefore, the person on a ketogenic diet consumes high amounts of fats, sufficient amounts of protein, and low amounts of carbs.

Normally, the body converts carbohydrates into glucose which it uses as an energy source. However, under ketosis, the body limits its intake of carbohydrates. This trigger the liver into breaking down fat cells, converting them into fatty acids and ketones, for use as an energy source later.

Just like any other diet, the ketogenic diet works by limiting the amount of calorie intake, generating a calorie shortage wherein your body burns more energy, than what it actually takes in. However, the key advantage of the ketogenic diet is its ability to help a person control his hunger way better than others in other diets. It can help you control your blood sugar and diminish the occurrence of an insulin spike.

When we consume a large amount of carbohydrate, our blood-glucose levels rise quickly. This also simultaneously produces rapid insulin response from our pancreatic gland, causing the dispersal of the excess blood glucose. As a result, we feel hungry all over again. In the ketogenic diet, you keep a low carbohydrate intake and because of this, you can maintain low blood sugar levels and avoid insulin spikes.

Remember that when you keep your insulin levels low, you also achieve dietary success, since it's the hormone that directs your body to accumulate fat.

You are able to create an environment in your body that reduces fat storage and encourages fat lipolysis. The ketogenic diet promotes satisfying meals in contrast with many diet plans which require the minimal intake of protein and fats. This allows you to continue enjoying various cuisines fused with both fat and protein. You'll realize how freeing carbohydrates and refined sugar will allow you to consume more satiating food in a day. According to many who observed the diet, they even have a hard time consuming an adequate amount of food daily.

Ketosis is a natural state wherein our body uses fats as the source of energy. Humans can use fats or carbohydrates as fuel. In consuming carbohydrates, your body automatically stores carbohydrates in muscles in the form of a substance called, "glycogen." Your body uses glycogen as its first option of fuel or energy source and any leftovers are finally stored as fats that contribute to weight gain.

Now, without glycogen as fuel, your body automatically uses its reserves, known as "fats." This process will force your body into the state of ketosis, making you limit your intake of carbohydrates and burning all the extra fat that you don't actually need. The state of ketosis isn't limited to your conscious activity but also occurs 'involuntarily' in your natural body function, making weight loss easy and certain to happen.

The idea of low carbohydrates, high fats, and sufficient protein intake is not an altogether new fad. It was introduced way back in the 1990's after the Dr. Atkins New Diet was released. Dr. Robert Atkins, the formulator of the Atkins Diet, discovered the benefits of ketosis in achieving weight loss for treating overweight 60-year old patients with heart diseases. Since then, the low-carb diet has become mainstream and has been adapted by various restaurants, offering low-carb diet options to their patrons.

People who observe the keto diet usually feel healthy, energetic and happy. They have smaller appetites and no sugary cravings, helping them lose weight. No need for them to use expensive specialist dietary products, instead they can enjoy appetizing protein and fat-based meals. In addition, a low-carb diet helps you to control your blood sugar since all sugars come from carbohydrates and all carbohydrates are eventually converted into sugars. With stable blood sugar levels, you no longer feel strong cravings for sugary foods, keeping blood sugar level fluctuations down and lower your risk of diseases like Type 2 diabetes.

The ketogenic diet works for weight loss program because of its effectiveness in using the body's natural behavior of burning off extra body fat without the side effects of feeling pangs of hunger, cravings and poor calorie intake. Additionally, people who practice ketogenic diet can lose weight without doing exercises, making it great for the obese, and people with injuries or disabilities.

Chapter 2: Advantages and Benefits of Ketogenic Diet

The ketogenic diet is embracing the idea of an extremely low carb diet to be in a state of ketosis. This state is simply burning fats as fuel instead of glucose. To achieve this state, deprive your body of the glucose through this diet plan and you can get some of these benefits:

Burns Fats Fast!

When you are in a ketosis, it allows your body to process fats quickly by using it as fuel in a way that no other state allows as easily. Because carbs are much easier to convert into energy vs fats, you need to burn and use it all before your body can start to convert fat into fuel. This is the reason why you tend to store fats in your body.

Harmless and Easy to Dispose

Ketones are not harmful to the body even when in excess. When your body produces so much that other ketones are no longer needed by the body, they are simply released through urination. You can be able to check every morning through the use of urine testing strips.

Bye, Bye to Sweet Tooth!

While your body gets used to being in a constant state of ketosis, it will prefer protein as a fuel source and will no longer crave for sugar. So, if you have a "sweet tooth", you'll be surprised to realize that you are no longer a glutton for sweets and desserts. This is because your system will actually prefer ketones over glucose.

Balance Insulin Level

While you are in a state of ketosis, it has the ability to control your insulin level. The primary purpose of insulin is to break down carbohydrates and convert them to glucose. It is likewise responsible for making you crave for sweets and starchy foods.

No More Cravings!

Being healthy is not based on the amount of food that you are taking in but rather on the food quality. Most people got into the habit of eating too much even when they don't need to eat, resulting to obesity. Obesity is one of the causes for many deadly illnesses.

Those who are into ketogenic diet testify that the diet indeed makes them significantly less hungry than when they were before. It is much easier to stick into a diet when you don't have to struggle against food cravings and hunger while on it. It's for these reasons that a person tend to lose his focus on his weight-loss goals. Therefore, if you don't have to deal with cravings, it is much easier to finish what you had started with your diet plan.

Chapter 3: Before Starting A Keto Diet, Know These Rules!

The ketogenic diet rules concentrate on eating little of carbs and protein, but lots of fat. It's not merely a diet which you can easily shift into and leave when another diet fad comes along. The ketogenic diet needs to be incorporated into your busy lifestyles, so you need to find out what will work best for you!

What to Eat

Generally, a keto diet consists of about 70-75% fat, 20-25% protein, and 5% carbs. These three macronutrients vary in their effects on ketosis depending on how they are digested and how they impact the glucose levels in the blood.

Carbohydrates cause the glucose and insulin levels to rise and is therefore 100% anti-ketogenic.

Protein is partly ketogenic and partly anti-ketogenic. More of protein consumed is converted to glucose that causes a rise in the insulin level.

Fat is 90% ketogenic and the remaining 10% anti-ketogenic. The anti-ketogenic element can convert triglycerides to glucose when the brain directs it to.

Fats effect on ketosis is minimal. The real impact is on how much weight you can lose as your body can either burn dietary fat or body fat as fuel.

Therefore, the more weight you want to lose, the more body fat you should burn. However, don't go overboard in limiting your fat intake as this will leave you hungrier and can be counter-productive. Knowing all these, always remember that ketogenic diets are very personal, and you must adopt one that works best for you.

Limit Carbohydrates

To start, don't eat more than 20 grams of net carbs each day. Over time you can up to 50 grams as most people should be able to remain in ketosis on a diet that contains up to 50 grams of net carbs.

Non-starchy vegetables must be your main source with more focus on green vegetables. Combine your carbohydrates with protein and fat.

Net Carbs

We count only net carbs. The objective here is to determine the actual impact any carb has on the blood sugar and insulin.

Carbs that are loaded with fiber and have much lower impact on blood sugars, which is why fibers are removed from the net carb calculation.

In fact, fiber does not convert into glucose like other carbs resulting in a lower glycemic load.

How Much Is Adequate Protein

Protein supports ketosis but too much of it will be converted into glucose. Therefore, it is surprising to hear people referring to ketogenic diet as a high-protein diet, which it is definitely not. Just take enough of protein to help protect muscle mass, but not beyond the required level so as not to disrupt ketosis. But how much is enough? How much is too much?

The amount of protein you need depends on how active you are. If you live a sedentary lifestyle, then you will only need about 0.7 -0.9 grams per grams per pound of lean body mass. As you become somewhat active, this will increase to about 0.0 to I gram per pound of lean body mass.

How to Calculate Lean Body Mass

Generally, lean body mass is calculated as total body weight minus body fat. There are many available online calculators if you want to calculate your lean body mass. As a general rule, men have a higher body mass than women and the average lean body mass is as follows:

- A healthy man's lean body mass is 76-84 percent.

- A healthy woman's lean body mass is 69-75 percent.

- Obese and overweight people have lower percentage.

How Much Protein Is Needed

Looking at these numbers, it is quite obvious that men need less protein than we actually thought. An inactive individual with a lean body mass of 150 pounds must eat 105-120 grams of protein per day. For an individual who is moderately active, the protein requirement will be between 120-150 grams and for a very active individual, it is 150-180.

Protein Choices

- Fatty red meats, chicken with its skin, turkey and deli meats

- Fish and seafood

- Eggs

- Full-fat dairy - heavy cream, sour cream, cheese

Some proteins like meat, poultry, and fish have zero net carbs, whilst overs like nuts and dairy have higher levels of net carbs and should be consumed in moderation.

Lots of Healthy Fats

Monounsaturated fats like olive oil and saturated fats like grass fed butter, red meat, and coconut oil are good fats.

Limit polyunsaturated fats like soybean, corn and cottonseed oil.

How much fat is needed by your body depends on your weight loss goal. As discussed previously, you need to consume 5 percent carbohydrates, 20-25 percent protein, and the good fat. To calculate your fat requirements, you need to work out on your daily calorie requirement based on your weight loss goal. From the total calories, subtract the carb and protein calories and the balance must be calories from fat.

Before you can calculate your fat requirement, you need to work out your daily calorie requirement which is based on your weight loss goal.

Chapter 4: What About Carbs?

Getting into a ketogenic diet can take some adjusting. While you have known all your life that fats in cheese and bacon are enemies when you want to lose weight, you would be greatly surprised to know when you look at the foods you can't eat on a ketogenic diet.

What is a Carbohydrate?

All carbohydrates are sugars. This can be surprising, especially if you think that foods you know as carbohydrates are not even sweet. Yes, not all carbohydrates are sweet but they are actually sugar. Sugars are simple carbohydrates and they make up sweet things like fructose – sugar that makes fruits deliciously sweet and enticing to the taste.

Starch and other complex carbohydrates including those found in bread, potatoes, rice pasta, root crops, and other high-carb foods, are actually made up of chains of sugar molecules. These are then broken down in your body by the enzyme called amylase that exists in your saliva and stomach so your body is able to digest carbohydrates as sugars.

Basically, food that contains sugar or starch contains carbohydrates, you need to count it towards your daily carb allowance on your keto diet. Foods that contain large quantities of carbohydrates must be avoided. This means all starchy fruits, rice, pastry, pasta and sweet vegetables like carrots and pepper must be avoided.

The Fiber's Role

There is this type of carbs that you are allowed to eat, and that is fiber. Fiber is easily digested by the body and the glucose from it won't enter your bloodstream. Once it passes through the body, it is largely unchanged, aiding your digestive system to move through other foods. Hence, when you calculate the carbs in a meal, you can subtract the fiber before adding it to your daily amount.

Chapter 5: Keto Recipes

You might have heard of famous celebrities observing the high-fat, low-carbohydrates diet—and they do have a good reason for doing so. With a low-carb diet, your body is nourished with whole foods, letting it burn fat as a source of energy and easily losing weight in the process.

This diet plan is perfect for those who have a busy life style!

- Very simple meal ideas with very little or no cooking required

- Meals you can easily take to eat at work

In this chapter, we are going to help you get started with designing your own ketogenic diet plan. We have provided sample recipes segregated into Breakfast, Lunch, Dinner meals. Of course, feel free switch between different meals or menu items at any time of the day. The 'breakfast' meals for instance, can easily double up as a quick lunch eaten on-to-go for the super busy.

Breakfast: Sausage, Spinach & Feta Frittata with a Cup of Coffee

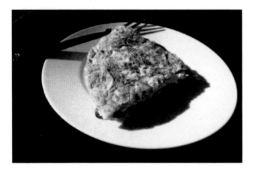

Ingredients

- 12 oz. of gluten-free mild pork sausage, roll

- 12 eggs

- 10 oz. package of frozen spinach, thawed and chopped

- ½ cup of plain and unsweetened almond milk

- ½ cup of feta cheese, crumbled

- ½ cup of heavy cream

- ¼ tsp. of ground nutmeg

- ¼ tsp. of black pepper

- ½ tsp. of salt

Directions

1. Break up the sausage into bits and put them in a medium-sized bowl.

2. Squeeze the extra liquid from the spinach and break the leaves into pieces. Put the bits into the same bowl as the sausage bits.

3. Sprinkle the mixture with feta cheese and lightly toss until they are mixed together.

4. Grease a 13x9 casserole dish or 18 muffin cups. Spread the mixture lightly onto the bottom of the dish or cups.

5. In a large bowl, combine the eggs, almond milk, heavy cream, nutmeg, salt, and pepper. Beat until they're incorporated well.

6. Pour into the dish (or muffin cups) until ¾ of the way full.

7. Bake at 375°F for about 50 minutes if you're using a casserole dish or half an hour if you're using muffin cups. Serve warm or at room temperature.

Note: This makes 18 muffins or 12 squares. For your diet, serve 3-inch square (1 pc. muffin) of this frittata together with a cup of coffee.

Nutrition Information:

- Per muffin: 137 calories, 10g fat, 8g protein, 1g net carbohydrates

- Per square: 206 calories, 16g fat, 12g protein, 1.4g net carbohydrates

- Coffee with 2tbsp. of heavy cream (120calories, 12g fat, 0.0g protein, 1g net carbohydrates

Breakfast: Cream Cheese Pancakes, Bacons, and Coffee

Ingredients

- 2 oz. of cream cheese
- 2 eggs
- ½ tsp. of cinnamon
- 1 tsp. of granulated sugar substitute

Directions

1. Place all the ingredients in a blender and process until you achieve a smooth consistency.
2. Let the mixture rest for about 2 minutes so that the bubbles can settle.
3. Heat a greased pan and pour a quarter of the batter into it. Cook for 2 minutes or until the side facing down is golden. Flip onto another side and cook for additional 1 minute. Repeat this step until you consume the rest of the batter.

Note: Serve 2 cream cheese pancakes along with 2 pieces of bacon. For the beverage, drink a cup of coffee with 2 tablespoons of heavy cream.

Nutrition Information:

- Cream cheese pancakes: 172 calories, 14g fat, 8g protein, 1g net carbohydrates

- Bacon: 92 calories, 7g fat, 6g protein, 0g net carbohydrates

- Coffee with heavy cream: 120 calories, 12g fat, 0g protein, 1g net carbohydrates

Breakfast: Ham & Cheese Frittata with a Cup of Coffee

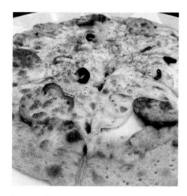

Ingredients

- 8 eggs
- ½ cup of deli ham, chopped
- ½ cup of mushrooms, chopped
- ½ cup of sharp cheddar cheese, shredded
- ¼ cup of heavy whipping cream
- ⅛ tsp. of ground nutmeg
- ¼ cup of fresh parsley, chopped
- 2 tbsp. of butter
- Salt
- Pepper

Directions

1. Melt butter and sauté the ham and mushrooms in a medium-sized, oven-proof pan.

2. Meanwhile, beat the eggs and cream together in a large bowl. Stir in the nutmeg then season with salt and pepper.

3. Pour the egg mixture over the ham and mushrooms. Gently mix in the cheese and the parsley.

4. Bake it at 375°F for 20-25 minutes or until it's firm. Serve with a cup of coffee.

Note: The recipe makes 6 servings.

Nutrition Information

- Ham & Cheese Frittata: 217 calories, 14g fat, 13g protein, 1g net carbohydrates

- Coffee with 2tbsp. of heavy cream: 120calories, 12g fat, 0g protein, 1g net carbohydrates

Breakfast: Monte Cristo Casserole with Poached Egg and Coffee

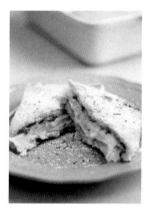

Ingredients

- 2 packages of 6.oz Canadian bacon

- 3 batches of cream cheese pancakes

- 1½ cups of Gruyere or Swiss cheese, shredded

- ⅓ cup of sugar-free pancake syrup, warmed

- To serve

- 1 egg, already poached

Directions

1. Prepare a 9x9 baking dish by greasing it with oil or cooking spray.

2. Assemble a layer of 4 cream cheese pancakes on the bottom and halfway up the sides of the dish. Add a layer of the bacon and top it with a half cup of cheese. Repeat this step until you make three layers.

3. Bake at 375°F for about 15 minutes or until it's completely heated through.

4. Remove the casserole from the oven. Pour syrup before topping it with the poached egg. Cut into 6 equal parts and serve with coffee. *Note:* The serving size of the casserole is 3.5 x 4-inch square.

Nutrition Information

- Monte Cristo Casserole: 376 calories, 24g fat, 32g protein, 4.5g net carbohydrates

- Poached egg: 80 calories, 6g fat, 6g protein, 0.5g net carbohydrates

- Coffee with 2tbsp. of heavy cream (120calories, 12g fat, 0g protein, 1g net carbohydrates

Breakfast: Inside-Out Scotch Eggs and Coffee

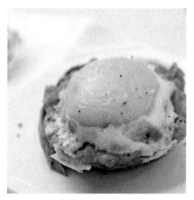

Ingredients

- 12 eggs

- 12 oz. of roll of ground Italian sausage

- Salt

- Pepper

- Avocado, sliced (or hot sauce)

Directions

1. Preheat oven to 375°F.

2. Divide the sausages into 12 one-ounce pieces proportional to the eggs. Place each piece into the muffin tins, observing half-inch thickness and about ¾ of the way up the sides then break one egg into each cup. (If you want your Scotch to be more of yolk, feel free to separate some of the white.)

3. Put your muffin tin on top of a cookie sheet to catch the grease from the sausage during the cooking process. Bake for about 18-22 minutes. Remove the Scotch eggs from the tins and season with salt and pepper.

4. Garnish with avocado slices or hot sauce. Serve with a cup of coffee

Note: 1 Scotch egg is equivalent to 1 serving.

Nutrition Information

- Scotch Eggs: 336 calories, 26g fat, 24g protein, 0.5g net carbohydrates

- Coffee with 2tbsp. of heavy cream: 120calories, 12g fat, 0g protein, 1g net carbohydrates

Breakfast: Cheesy Italian Omelette with a Cup of Coffee

Ingredients

- 2 eggs
- 3 thin slices of deli Sopressata (salami or prosciutto)
- 2 oz. fresh mozzarella cheese
- 5 thin slices fresh, ripe tomato
- 6 fresh basil leaves
- 1 tbsp. of butter
- 1 tbsp. of water
- Salt
- Pepper

Directions

1. In a small bowl, whisk the eggs and water together.

2. Place a nonstick pan over medium heat and melt the butter. Pour in the egg mixture and cook for half a minute.

3. Spread the meat slices on the one-half side of the egg. Top with tomatoes, cheese, and basil, then season with salt and pepper. Cook for about 2 minutes or until the other half—the empty one—is firm enough to fold over the ingredients. In folding, use a spatula to put the empty side over the other half.

4. Cover the pan and continue to cook on low heat for another minute or until the omelet is cooked through.

5. To serve, tilt the pan and let the omelet gently slide onto your serving plate. Serve with a cup of coffee.

Note: This recipe makes one generous serving of omelet.

Nutrition Information

- Cheesy Italian Omelette: 451 calories, 36g fat, 33g protein, 3g net carbohydrates

- Coffee with 2tbsp. of heavy cream: 120 calories, 12g fat, 0g protein, 1g net carbohydrates

Breakfast: Blackberry Egg Bake and Coffee

Ingredients

- ½ cup of fresh blackberries
- 5 large eggs
- 3 tbsp. of coconut flour
- 1 tbsp. of butter, melted
- 1 tsp. of fresh ginger, grated
- 1 tsp. of fresh rosemary, finely chopped
- ¼ tsp. of vanilla
- zest of half an orange
- ⅓ tsp. of fine sea salt

Directions

1. Preheat oven to 350°F and grease 4 ramekins.
2. Put all the ingredients together (except for the blackberries and rosemary) into a blender and blend on high for about 1-2 minutes or until you achieved a smooth consistency. Add the rosemary and pulse for several times until the rosemary is mixed completely with the mixture.
3. Divide the mixture proportionate to the 4 ramekins. Distribute the berries to each ramekin as well.
4. Put the ramekins on a baking sheet and bake for about 15-20 minutes until the egg mixture is cooked through. Let them cool on a rack before serving. Serve with a cup of coffee per serving.

Note: This recipe makes 4 servings. 1 ramekin is equivalent to 1 serving.

Nutrition Information

- Blackberry Egg Bake: 144 calories, 10g fat, 8.5g protein, 2g net carbohydrates
- Coffee with 2tbsp. of heavy cream: 120 calories, 12g fat, 0g protein, 1g net carbohydrates

Lunch: Green Enchilada Meatballs

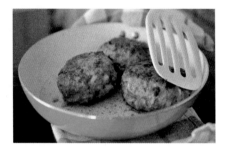

Ingredients

- 1 lb. of ground chicken or turkey
- ¼ cup of almond flour
- ¼ cup of queso fresco, crumbled
- 1 egg
- 2 tbsp. of green onions, chopped
- 1 tbsp. of ground cumin
- 1 tbsp. ground coriander
- 1 tbsp. of cilantro, chopped
- 1 tsp. garlic powder
- ½ tsp. of salt
- ¼ tsp black pepper
- Oil, enough for frying

To serve

- ½ cup of salsa verde
- ¼ cup of queso fresco, crumbled

Instructions

1. Thoroughly mix all the ingredients in a medium-size bowl and form 16 meatballs.

2. Heat oil in a large, non-stick pan and cook the meatballs for 3-4 minutes on each side. Remove and set aside.

3. To serve, spread a few tablespoons of salsa berde on the bottom of a large serving dish. Assemble the meatballs on top of the salsa and pour the remaining over each meatball. Sprinkle with queso fresco on top and serve immediately.

Note: Four meatballs is equal to one serving.

Nutrition Information

- 341 calories, 28g fat, 32g protein, 3.5g net carbohydrates

Lunch: Simple Egg Salad with Bacon and Lettuce

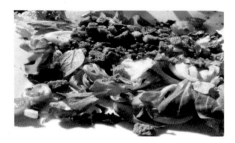

Ingredients

- 6 eggs

- 2 tbsp. of mayonnaise

- 1 tsp. of lemon juice

- 1 tsp. of Dijon mustard

- ¼ tsp. of lite salt

- Kosher salt

- Pepper

- 4 Romaine lettuce leaves

- 2 slices of bacon

Directions

1. Boil the eggs for about 10 minutes, remove from heat and set aside to cool.

2. Peel the eggs and process in a food processor until they're chopped.

3. Add the mayonnaise, lemon juice, mustard, pepper plus the lite and kosher salts.

4. Serve with lettuce leaves and bacon.

Nutrition Information

*   262 calories, 21g fat, 16g protein, 1g net carbohydrates

Lunch: Meatballs Alla Parmigiana

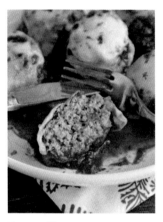

Ingredients

For the meatballs

- 1.5 lbs. of ground beef (80/20)
- 2 eggs
- ½ cup of almond flour
- 2 tbsp. of fresh parsley, chopped
- ¾ cup of parmesan cheese, grated
- ¼ tsp. of dried oregano
- ¼ tsp. of garlic powder
- 1 tsp. of dried onion flakes
- ½ cup of warm water
- 1 tsp. of kosher salt
- ¼ tsp. of ground black pepper

For the Parmigiana:

- 1 cup of marinara sauce
- 4 oz. of mozzarella cheese

Directions

1. In a large mixing bowl, incorporate all the meatball ingredients and mix well.

2. Make 15 pieces of 2-inch meatballs.

3. You can either bake them at 350°F for about 20 minutes or fry them in a large skillet over medium flame.

4. For the parmigiana, place all the meatballs in an oven-safe dish. Pour at least 1 tbsp. of sauce over each meatball. Cover them with mozzarella cheese and bake for another 20 minutes at 350°F or until the cheese is golden.

5. Garnish with parsley and serve.

Note: This recipe makes 15 meatballs. For one serving, serve 3 meatballs.

Nutrition Information

- 453 calories, 27g fat, 36g protein, 5g net carbohydrates

Lunch: Southern Fried Chicken with Baby Spinach

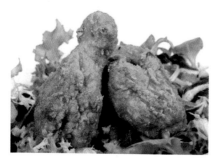

Ingredients

- 5 lbs. of chicken leg quarters
- 1 cup of coconut flour
- 1 tsp. of paprika
- 1 tsp. of garlic powder
- 1 tsp. of salt
- 1 tsp. of pepper
- Oil, for frying

Directions

1. Combine the chicken, garlic powder, paprika, salt and pepper in a large bowl. Massage the spices to the chicken until it's well coated. Cover the bowl and refrigerate for 2 hours (or overnight if you want it to be more flavorful).

2. To cook, add the coconut flour and mix to coat well. Heat 2-inch deep oil in a large skillet (or deep fryer) to 375°F.

3. Cook the chicken in batches for 8 minutes per side or until it's golden brown. If you want them to be crisp, don't overcrowd your pan. Use a meat thermometer to know if the internal temperature reaches 165°F. Alternatively, you can cut the meat to make sure that it's no longer pink.

4. Serve with 2 cups of raw baby spinach together dressed with 1 tbsp. of sugar-free ranch dressing.

Note: This recipe makes 6 servings.

Nutrition Information

- Southern Fried Chicken: 425 calories, 32g fat, 34g protein, 1g net carbohydrates

- Baby Spinach: 14 calories, 0g fat, 2g protein, 1g net carbohydrates

- Ranch Dressing: 70 calories, 7g fat, 0g protein, 1g net carbohydrates

Lunch: Salmon Patties with Fresh Herbs

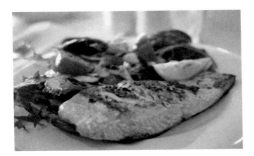

Ingredients

- 2 x 4.75-oz. cans of pink salmon, drained
- ½ cup almond flour
- 2 large eggs
- 4 oz. pork rinds, crushed
- ¼ cup of Parmesan cheese, grated
- ¼ cup of fresh dill, chopped
- 2 tbsp. of fresh chives, chopped
- 1 tsp. of lemon zest
- 2 tbsp. of olive oil
- Salt
- Pepper

Directions

1. In a large bowl, combine the salmon, eggs, parmesan, chives, dill, pork rinds, lemon zest, salt, and pepper. Make 10 3-ounce balls from the mixture.

2. Put the almond flour in a plate and proceed into flattening each patty using the palm of your hands. Dip each patty into the flour but make sure that the patties do not break.

3. Place skillet over medium-high heat and add 2 tbsp. of oil. Cook the patties until both sides are browned.

4. Serve with 2 cups of baby spinach and a tablespoon of sugar-free ranch dressing.

Note: This recipe makes 5 servings. 2 patties make one serving.

Nutrition Information

-   Salmon patties: 418 calories, 25g fats, 46g protein, 2.63g net carbohydrates

-   Baby Spinach: 14 calories, 0g fat, 2g protein, 1g net carbohydrates

-   Ranch Dressing: 70 calories, 7g fat, 0g protein, 1g net carbohydrates

Lunch: Avgolemeno Soup and Keto Muffin

Avgolemeno Soup

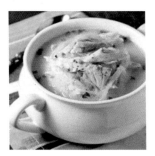

Ingredients

- 10 cups of chicken stock or broth

- 4 cups of chicken, cooked and shredded

- 3 eggs

- 2 cups of spaghetti squash, cooked

- ¼ cup of fresh parsley, chopped

- ⅓ cup of fresh lemon juice

- Salt

- Pepper

- Parmesan cheese, freshly grated

Directions

1. In a large saucepan, bring the broth and chicken to a boil. Once it boils, remove from the heat.

2. Whisk the eggs and the lemon juice together in a medium-size bowl until frothy. Gently whisk in 2 cups of hot stock into the egg mixture (don't just pour it in as you will end up with scrambled eggs).

3. Once the stock has been fully combined into the egg mixture, pour this back into the saucepan. Add the spaghetti squash and reheat if necessary (just use low heat so that the egg won't curdle).

4. Season with salt and pepper. Garnish with parmesan cheese and parsley before serving.

Note: This recipe makes 8 servings. 1 ½ cups of this soup is equivalent to one serving.

Keto Muffin

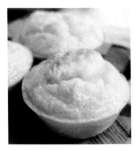

Ingredients

- 1 large egg
- 2 tsp. of coconut flour
- A pinch of baking soda
- A pinch of salt

Directions

1. Prepare a ramekin dish by greasing it with coconut oil or butter.
2. Combine all the ingredients together in a microwave-safe mug. Use a fork to make sure that there will be no lumps.
3. Transfer the dough into the ramekin and microwave on high temperature for 1 minute. If you're using an oven, put it on 400°F about 12 minutes.
4. Cut in half before serving.

Note: This recipe is good for one serving only.

Nutrition Information

- Avgolemeno Soup: 289 calories, 15g fat, 33g protein, 4g net carbohydrates

- Keto muffin: 202 calories, 18g fat, 7g protein, 3g net carbohydrates

Dinner: Rotisserie Chicken with Cauliflower Gratin

Ingredients

- 4 cups of raw cauliflower florets
- 6 deli slices pepper jack cheese
- 4 tbsp. of butter
- ⅓ cup of heavy whipping cream
- Salt
- Pepper

Directions

1. Combine the cauliflower, cream, butter, salt, and pepper in a microwave-safe dish and mix well.

2. Microwave the mixture on high for about 10- 25 minutes (depending on how you can easily cook the cauliflower) or until the cauliflower is tender. The key here is to make the vegetable soft until you can easily mash it with a fork.

3. Remove the dish from the microwave and proceed to mash the cauliflower.

4. Season with salt and pepper if so desired.

5. Set the cheese slices across the top of the cauliflower and microwave for another 2-3 minutes. Serve hot.

Note: Serve a ¾ cup of cauliflower gratin with 6 oz. rotisserie chicken, 2 cups of chopped Romaine lettuce and 2 tbs. of sugar-free Caesar salad dressing.

Nutrition Information

1. Rotisserie chicken: 276 calories, 11g fat, 42g protein, 0g net carbohydrates

2. Cauliflower Gratin: 215 calories, 19g fat, 6g protein, 2g net carbohydrates

3. Romaine lettuce: 16 calories, 0g fat, 1g protein, 1g net carbohydrates

4. Caesar Salad Dressing: 170 calories, 18g fat, 1g protein, 2g net carbohydrates

Dinner: Paprika Chicken and Cheesy Cauliflower Puree

Paprika Chicken

Ingredients

- 4 large chicken thighs, with bone in and skin on

- ¼ cup sour cream

- 2 tbsp. of Hungarian Paprika

- 1 tsp. of onion powder

- 1 tsp. of kosher salt

Directions

1. In a small bowl, combine the onion powder, paprika and kosher salt together.

2. Season the chicken thighs with the mixture and place on a baking sheet lined with parchment paper.

3. Roast the thighs at 400°F for 40 minutes.

4. Transfer the chicken to a plate and pour the juices into the sheet into a small bowl. Add the sour cream into the bowl until you achieve a smooth consistency.

5. Serve the chicken together with the gravy.

Note: This recipe makes 4 servings. One chicken thigh is equivalent to 1 serving.

Cheesy Cauliflower Puree

Ingredients

- 1 head of cauliflower, clean, trimmed and broken into medium-size pieces
- 2 oz. of Dubliner or any other sharp cheese
- 2 tsp. of heavy cream
- 1 tsp. of butter
- Salt
- Pepper

Instructions

1. Put the cauliflower into a microwave-safe bowl. Add the cream and butter.

2. Microwave, uncovered, on high for about 6 minutes. Mix to coat the cauliflower with the butter-cream mixture then microwave again for another 6 minutes on high.

3. Remove from the microwave and transfer to a blender or food processor together with the cheese. Process this until you achieve the consistency of a puree.

4. Season with salt and pepper. Serve.

Note: Serve the puree together with 2 cups of chopped Romaine lettuce dressed with 2 tbsp. of sugar-free Italian dressing.

Nutrition Information

- Paprika Chicken: 384 calories, 31g fat, 33g protein, 1g net carbohydrates

- Cheesy Cauliflower Puree: 148 calories, 11g fat, 6g protein, 4g net carbohydrates

- Romaine Lettuce with dressing: 86 calories, 6g fat, 1g protein, 1g net carbohydrates

Dinner: Sausage-Veggie Soup and Jalapeno & Cheddar Muffin

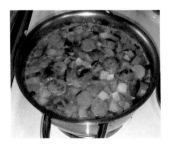

Sausage-Veggie Soup

Ingredients

- 1 lb. of sweet Italian turkey sausage
- 4 cups of kale, chopped
- 3 cups of pumpkin or butternut squash, chopped
- ½ cup of onion, chopped
- 4 cups of chicken broth
- 4 cups of water

For garnish

- Parmesan cheese, grated
- Red pepper flakes, crushed

Directions

1. In a medium saucepan, cook the sausage according to package instruction. Once cooked, add the onions and saute until it turns translucent. Add both water and chicken broth and bring to boil.

2. Reduce the heat before adding the pumpkin and kale. Let it simmer for about 20 minutes or until the pumpkin is already soft.

3. Garnish with parmesan and red pepper flakes.

Note: This recipe makes 8 servings; 1 ¾ cup makes one serving.

Jalapeno & Cheddar Muffin

Ingredients

- 2 cups of raw cauliflower, finely diced
- 2 eggs, beaten
- 1 cup of cheddar cheese, grated
- 1 cup of mozzarella cheese, grated
- ⅓ cup of parmesan cheese, grated
- ¼ cup of coconut flour
- 2 tbsp. of jalapeno, minced
- 2 tbsp. of butter, melted
- 1 tbsp. of dried onion flakes
- ½ tsp. of garlic powder
- ½ tsp. of baking powder
- ¼ tsp. of salt
- ¼ tsp. of black pepper

Directions

1. Preheat oven to 375°F.

2. In a medium bowl, mix all jalapeno, eggs, melted butter and cauliflower. Add mozzarella, parmesan, and cheddar and mix well. Add the coconut flour, baking powder, onion flakes, garlic powder, salt, and pepper. Stir the mixture well until everything is well combined.

3. Pour the butter into 12 greased muffin cups, dividing them equally among the cups.

4. Bake for half an hour or until the muffins are golden brown. Turn off the oven and leave them inside for another 1 hour. Serve warm or cold.

Nutrition Information

- Sausage- Veggie Soup: 118 calories, 6g fat, 11g protein, 5.5g net carbohydrates

- Jalapeno & Cheddar Muffin: 110 calories, 8g fat, 8g protein, 2g net carbohydrate

Dinner: Cajun Chicken-Stuffed Avocado

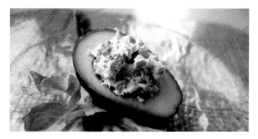

Ingredients

- 1 extra large or 2 medium avocados, seed removed
- 1 ½ of cup chicken, cooked and shredded
- 2 tbsp. of fresh lemon juice
- ¼ cup of mayonnaise
- 2 tbsp. of sour cream or cream cheese
- 1 tsp. of paprika
- 1 tsp. of thyme, dried
- ¼ tsp. of cayenne pepper
- ½ tsp. of onion powder
- ½ tsp. of garlic powder
- ¼ tsp. of salt

Directions

1. In a medium bowl, combine the chicken, sour cream (or cream cheese), mayonnaise, paprika, thyme, cayenne, lemon juice, onion powder, garlic powder, and salt. Mix together until combined well.

2. Scoop the middle of the avocado, leaving half to one inch of its flesh.

3. Chop the scooped out avocado flesh and put them into the chicken mixture. Mix until completely combined.

4. Scoop chicken-avocado mixture into the middle of the avocado, filling all four avocado halves, and serve.

Note: This recipe makes 2 servings.

Nutrition Information

- 638 calories, 50.6g fat, 34.5g protein, 5.4g net carbohydrates

Dinner: Low-Carb Chili

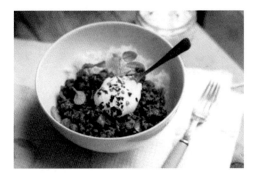

Ingredients

- 1 lb. of lean ground beef (or turkey)
- ½ cup of prepared salsa
- ½ tsp. of ground cayenne
- ½ tsp. of garlic powder
- 1 tsp. of ground coriander
- 1 tsp. of ground cumin
- Salt
- Pepper

For garnish

- 2 tbsp. of sour cream
- 1 tbsp. of cilantro, chopped
- ¼ cup of cheddar cheese, shredded

Directions

1. Combine the beef (or turkey) and all the spices in a medium-size saucepan. Place over medium heat and let the meat be cooked through. Add the salsa and let it simmer for about 5 minutes.

2. Garnish with cheese, sour cream and cilantro.

Note: This recipe makes 4 servings.

Nutrition Information

- 394 calories, 23g of fat, 41g protein, 3.75g net carbohydrates

Dinner: Brazilian Shrimp Stew

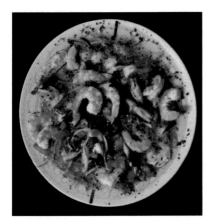

Ingredients

- 1½ lbs. of raw shrimp, peeled and deveined
- 14 oz.- can of diced tomatoes with chilis
- 1 cup of coconut milk
- ¼ cup of olive oil
- ¼ cup of onion, diced
- 1 clove of garlic, minced
- ¼ cup of roasted red pepper, diced
- ¼ cup of fresh cilantro, chopped
- 2 tbsp. of Sriracha hot sauce
- 2 tbsp. of fresh lime juice
- Salt
- Pepper

Directions

1. In a medium-size saucepan, heat olive oil and sauté onions until translucent. Add garlic and peppers. Continue to sauté for several minutes. Add the shrimp, tomatoes, and cilantro. Let it simmer until the shrimp turns opaque.

2. Next, pour in the Sriracha sauce and coconut milk. Cook until it's heated through but remember not to bring it to a boil. Add the lime juice and season with salt and pepper. Garnish with cilantro and serve.

Note: This recipe makes 6 servings. 1 cup is equivalent to one serving.

Nutrition Information

- 294 calories, 19g fat, 24g protein, 5g net carbohydrates

Dinner: Bacon & Smoked Gouda Cauliflower Mash

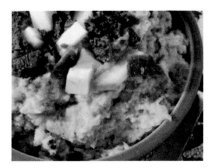

Ingredients

- 4 slices of cooked bacon
- 4 cups of cauliflower florets
- ⅓ cup Smoked Gouda cheese, shredded
- 3 tbsp. of heavy cream
- 2 tbsp. of butter
- ¼ tsp. of garlic powder
- ½ tsp. of kosher salt
- ¼ tsp. of black pepper
- Salt
- Pepper

Directions

1. In a microwave-safe dish, put the cauliflower, butter, garlic powder, heavy cream, kosher salt, and pepper. Microwave on high temperature for about 18-20 minutes or until tender.

2. Transfer the cauliflower mixture to a food processor then add the bacon and Gouda. Process until you achieve a smooth and creamy consistency. If you want, you can season with additional salt and pepper.

Note: This recipe makes 3 cups. 1 cup is equivalent to 1 serving.

Cajun Chicken

Ingredients

- 5 lbs. of chicken thighs
- ¼ cup Cajun seasoning
- 2 tbsp. of olive oil

To serve

- Ranch dressing

Directions

1. Preheat oven to 400°F.
2. Massage the chicken with olive oil, then add the Cajun seasoning. Toss until the chicken is completely coated. Place the chicken on a cooking sheet (or cooking sheets), observing 1-inch spaces between each piece.
3. Bake for about 50 minutes or until the skin is all golden and crispy.

Note: This recipe makes 6-8 servings. 2 pieces of thighs make 1 serving.

Nutrition Information

- Bacon & Gouda Cauliflower Mash: 282 calories, 22g fat, 12g protein, 6g net carbohydrates

- Cajun Chicken: 495 calories, 26g fat, 60g protein, 0 net carbohydrates

Dinner: Roasted Chicken & Tomatoes with Wilted Beet Green Salad

Roasted Chicken & Tomatoes

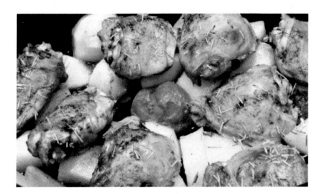

Ingredients

- 4 large Roma tomatoes, washed and halved

- 4 large chicken thighs or wings

- 2 tbsp. of olive oil

- 1 tbsp. of fresh thyme

- Salt

- Pepper

Directions

1. Put all the chicken thighs and the tomatoes (with the cut side up) in a baking dish. Season with salt and pepper, then drizzle with olive oil. Sprinkle with fresh thyme before roasting at 375°F for about an hour.

Note: Serving size is 1 chicken thigh and 2 tomato halves.

Wilted Beet Green Salad

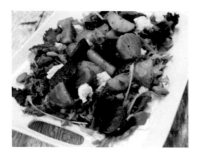

Ingredients

- 4 cups of beet greens, washed and chopped
- 3 tsp. of olive oil
- 2 tbsp. of pine nuts, toasted
- 1 tbsp. of balsamic vinegar (no sugar added)

Directions

- Heat one tsp. of olive oil in a large skillet and sauté the beet greens for about 4 minutes or until they're tender. Get the skillet off the heat and season the greens with salt and pepper.

- Meanwhile, mix the vinegar and 2 tbsp. of olive oil using a fork.

- Before serving, garnish the greens with goat cheese and pine nuts. Finally, drizzle with the vinegar-oil mixture. Serve with the roasted chicken and tomatoes.

Note: This recipe makes 2 generous servings.

Nutrition Information

- Roasted Chicken & Tomatoes: 409 calories, 28g fat, 36g protein, 1.5g net carbohydrates

- Wilted Beet Green Salad: 215 calories, 18g fat, 10g protein, 3.5g net carbohydrates

Chapter 6: Exercises and Keto Diet

You must have read somewhere that a Ketogenic Diet is one of the safest ways to lose weight without exercising. It has been said that one of the best things about following a keto diet is that you don't have to adopt an exercise regime to lose weight. Many people dislike the idea of working out, or think they lack time, and this makes the ketogenic diet so appealing. This is quite true! When your body is in a state of ketosis, it is constantly burning up fats, making you lose weight even when you aren't moving much. Your body's stored fat is being used up when you don't have enough carbohydrates to fuel up your body.

However, it doesn't mean that you can't or won't need to exercise when you're on a ketogenic diet plan. You need to adopt an exercise regimen alongside your ketogenic diet, if you want to achieve faster and more effective weight loss results.

This is because of how a ketogenic diet works. Since you are always burning fat in ketosis, the entire energy burn of your workout is coming from your fat stores. If you have a carbohydrate rich diet, it takes around twenty minutes of cardio or aerobic work before you can get into that "fat burning zone". On a low carb diet, you're burning it right from the get go!

Additionally, because a ketogenic diet only burns fat, and doesn't cause you to lose lean muscle like a severely low-calorie diet, the effects of any muscle building or toning exercise will be more pronounced. The fat will strip off, revealing those lean, strong muscles – but only if you work on them. This means that a ketogenic diet and exercise when used together will give you a leaner and toner body.

If you are new to exercise, overweight or recovering from an injury, start with 30 minutes of easy cardio like brisk walking, or swimming. Do this three times a week and add some resistance training for lean muscle mass improvement. As you become lighter in weight and with your body getting fitter, you can then increase the intensity of your workouts.

Workouts are generally divided into three types: aerobic, anaerobic, and stability.

Aerobic exercise, also known as cardio exercise. Lower intensity, steady-state cardio is fat burning, making it very friendly for the keto dieter.

Examples: 30-minute runs, swims, bike rides, spinning

Anaerobic exercise is characterized by shorter bursts of energy, such as weight training or high-intensity interval training (HIIT). Carbohydrates are the primary fuel for anaerobic exercise, so fat alone can't provide enough energy for this type of workout.

Stability exercises include balance exercises and core training. They help improve your alignment, strength muscles, and control of movement. Examples: abdominal or isometric exercises.

As you exercise regularly and get fitter, you will begin to find that it's getting hard for you to perform as compared to earlier exercises because of the absence of glycogen in your body. As soon as you feel this, you can switch to a targeted or cyclical diet plan, so you can have enough carbs to get you through higher impact workouts.

A cyclical ketogenic diet plan means that you load your body with carbohydrates on weekends but for the rest of the week, you need to go back to a low carb diet. In a targeted ketogenic diet plan, you are allowed to eat some extra carbs before your workout.

For Beginners

Slow cardio is easily the best type of exercise for the keto dieter. And most people should begin with a cardio program first.

However, if you have been training hard for several weeks with no significant effect on your weight loss, realize that only using cardio for your fat loss may not be a sustainable lifestyle for you. Everyone's metabolism or physiology make-up is different. If you are still not losing weight, but are instead experiencing the following, it's time to switch workouts!

1. Repetitive or prolonged cardio will make you even hungrier and more likely to eat more. Your body wants to replace those lost calories!

2. Intense cardio increases the stress hormone, cortisol, responsible to storing visceral fats in the tummy area.

3. Inflammation from over-training or over-use, leading to pain or strain in your musculoskeletal structure. E.g. constant running may lead to tendon or joint strain in your legs.

For Advanced

The best exercise program uses a combination of different exercises, sometimes on different days, among aerobic, anaerobic, and stability exercises. Even doing a cardio workout, it's best to switch exercises from time to time to avoid musculoskeletal strain e.g switching from runs to swims on some days.

For the more experienced, begin strength/resistance training) and high-intensity interval training. For ladies, don't worry about getting bulky, a woman's body simply don't have the hormones to get 'muscular'. Putting on muscles is not as easy as many people think, and especially if you are a woman.

HIIT or High Intensity Interval Training is easily one of the best for prolonged weight loss.

What is interval training? It's a training technique in which you alternate intense bursts of anaerobic exercise such as sprinting or calisthenics with short recovery periods. One of the effects is that you burn more calories in less time compared to other workouts like prolonged cardio.

My sample HIIT workout, in sequence, rest as little as possible.

1. Pull-ups

2. Push-ups

3. Dips

4. Squats

5. Lunges

6. Sprints

You can of course modify the exercises to suit the location, your preferences or ability levels. The beauty of my HIIT sequence is that it is simple, can be done anywhere outdoors, and take up as little time as possible, while triggering the highest fat burn and boosting your metabolism level for hours.

For The Dedicated

Day 1

Gym workout or HIIT day. Lift in short, intense sessions. Resistance training provides numerous benefits, including muscle gain and fat loss. Focus on anaerobic and stability work. Session should be short and intense, with as few breaks as possible. Time spend should not exceed 1 hour.

Day 3

Gym or strength train using lower-repetition sets. Keep your sets to 10 reps or less, and if this means you need to increase the weight, still select a weight that you can safely control. If you want more volume, perform more sets. This will allow your depleted glycogen, or sugar reserves to replenish slightly between sets.

Day 5

Perform intense cardio exercise. However, a note of caution, long endurance sessions may be difficult if don't have enough carbs in you. Example, if you wish to run three miles, but the lack of carbohydrates limits your performance, run your distance in interval fashion. Run as far as you can, walk until you recover, then continue at your run pace. This can be duplicated for any form of cardio exercise.

Post Workout

Eat a small amount of carbohydrates post-workout. Following your workout, your blood sugar is extremely low and your body will shuttle sugars you consume directly to your muscles. This will help refill the muscle glycogen that you burned during training.

Tips

Consume a small amount of whey protein with your carbohydrates following a workout. In addition to burning sugar, your body will also break down amino acids during training.

You can load up on carbs over the weekend if you follow a cyclical ketogenic diet

Conclusion

Getting into the Ketogenic Diet is never easy. When you embrace the diet plan, you will not only be dealing with the tough mental discipline it required, but you need to cope with all the physiological challenges it brings. Maintaining your emotional perseverance can be tough at times because so many distractions and social pressures may derail your best efforts. Keep the ultimate end goal in mind – to craft a lean, slim, and healthy body, and anything is possible.

-- Rick Elliott

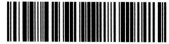

79869251R00038

Made in the USA
Middletown, DE
12 July 2018